INTRODUCTION

If you are reading this book, you most likely have already started a church or ministry and now you want to sure that you have set it up properly, or you are on verge of starting an incredible journey. In either case, this is the book for you.

I have spent the bulk of my career, both as a lawyer and as an executive, working at the intersection of faith and business. This book is a reflection of that. My personal mission – my WHY?, if you will, is to enable those passionate people who have made a decision to follow God's call on their life and dare to make an impact on the world.

This book meets that objective by providing you, the visionary, with a straightforward, easy to understand guide for structuring and establishing a non-profit corporation for your church or ministry. If you are just starting out, this book will get you started on the right foot. If you have been operating for a while (even years), this book will help you get on the right track to protect you and your organization.

Essentially, this book is a guide to building a solid legal foundation for your ministry that can withstand the weight that will follow with success.

What is a corporation and why do I need one?

The moment has come. You have decided that the season has arrived and it is time for you to start a new church or ministry. You know what God wants you to do. The question is, "What do you do next?" From a legal perspective, the answer is easy; you need to form a non-profit corporation through which you will operate you church or ministry.

A corporation is simply an entity that the law has created so that a group of people can operate a common enterprise together for a common objective. The law allows people to form an entity, called a corporation, so that the enterprise – be it a church, oil company or car wash – can have its own existence separate and apart from the people who operate the enterprise.

This separate existence provides a corporation with two distinct advantages. First, a corporation will provide you with personal legal protection against liability. Because the corporation has a separate legal existence from the people who run it, as a general matter, the corporation, not the people who operate the corporation, is accountable for the actions of the corporation. In other words, the corporation acts as a legal shield of protection for the individuals involved in running the church.

Here is a quick example. Assume that the church bus is involved in an accident and that the accident was caused by Elder Brown, a church employee, and that Bob Jones, the driver of the other vehicle involved in the accident is seriously injured and incurs several thousand dollars in medical bills and is off work for six months. Bob Jones is going to want somebody to pay. Without the protection of a corporation, Pastor Wilson who runs the church, but who was nowhere near the accident, is likely to be the one who gets sued by Bob Jones. If a corporation exists, it will be the corporation that gets sued, not the individual.

Similar rules apply to the debts and obligations of the church. If the corporation incurred the debts, the corporation alone is liable for those debts (unless some individual personally guaranteed the debt). Clearly, the separate existence and legal shield afforded by forming a corporation are extremely beneficial.

Moreover, forming a non-profit corporation will make it much easier for your church to enjoy the advantages of being tax-exempt. While it is possible for a church to operate on a tax-exempt basis without forming a corporation (a church that operates without being incorporated is an unincorporated association), it is often difficult. Businesses and governmental agencies particularly are used to dealing with corporate entities. Forming a non-profit corporation makes it very clear what your organization is and is not. As a result, filing for and obtaining various exemptions for sales taxes, property taxes and the like will be greatly eased.

In the last paragraph, I used the term "non-profit corporation". Before we move on to how to structure and form a non-profit corporation, let me take a quick moment to distinguish between the different types of corporations. Most of us are familiar with a regular corporation which is a for-profit entity. Millions of businesses, large and small, are organized as regular for-profit corporations. These organizations are owned by individuals (or other entities) called shareholders. The shareholders reap the financial rewards of "owning" the corporation. Non-profit corporations, on the other hand, are operated for the public good and are not "owned" by anyone. When a non-profit corporation earns a "profit" at the end of the year (yes, a non-profit can and should earn a "profit" if it is going to stay in existence and grow), the money does not go to shareholders (there are no shareholders). Instead, the funds generated by the non-profit must be used for the exempt purposes for which corporation was formed (such as charitable, educational, religious – more about this later).

In essence, our local, state and federal governments have made a deal. The deal is that in exchange for the tax-exempt status that is granted to most non-profits (yes it is possible to be a non-profit, but taxable corporation – more about this later), non-profits cannot be owned by any individual. Instead, the earnings of the organization (including the savings that result from not having to pay taxes) must be used for an allowed purpose that the government has determined benefits society in general (such as educational, charitable, and religious purposes).

The implication of this concept is immense. Because no one, not even the founder of a church or ministry, owns any part of the non-profit corporation, no one should conduct themselves as if they do own it. The corporation exists for the public benefit and should be treated as such. This means that the corporation's assets cannot be used as if they belong to an individual. A non-profit corporation cannot freely distribute its assets to people. It can only pay fair value for goods and services received. This means its employees can earn a reasonable salary and benefits in exchange for their efforts, but that it is it (again, more about this later).

Why then, would you form a non-profit corporation instead of a for-profit corporation? The answer is simple, tax and donations. Most non-profits, including all churches are exempt from most taxes such as property, sales and income taxes. Moreover, non-profits can receive donations and the donors can take a tax deduction for the amount of the donation.

In other words, the government has chosen to give up billions in tax revenue, but the trade-off is that non-profit corporations have to be operated for the benefit of the public, not individuals. So when you complain about the regulations imposed on churches and other non-profits, remember the deal. You can get rid of the regulation anytime you want to, as long as you are ready to pay the tax and give up the donations.

The bottom-line is that, if you have not already done so, you need to establish a non-profit corporation through which you will operate your church or ministry.

Steps to forming a non-profit corporation

Today, the actual process of forming a non-profit corporation is a relatively quick and simple four-step process. Once a few key decisions have been made, most lawyers (or non-lawyers with the aid of online services) can complete the paperwork in a relatively short time. The steps are follows:

1. Articles of Incorporation (also called a Certificate of Incorporation or Certificate of Formation in some states) are prepared and filed with the designated state official, typically the Secretary of State in your state (or the state where you want to incorporate) and the required filing fee is paid. Once the Secretary of State has accepted the Articles for filing, the corporation begins to exist as a separate entity.

2. An initial meeting of the Board of Directors of the newly formed corporation must be held to (i) approve its formation, (ii) adopt Bylaws (sometimes referred to as a "Constitution"), (iii) elect officers to run the corporation and take care of a few other housekeeping matters. This meeting can be held either in person or by written consent signed by all of the Board members (how I usually do this).

3. The corporation needs to apply for and receive a Tax ID Number (also called an EIN or Employer Identification Number). This is effectively the social security number for the corporation. The Tax ID Number can be obtained online at www.irs.gov in a few minutes.

4. Armed with a copy of the corporation's Articles, Bylaws and Tax ID Number, you can go to your bank and open a bank account in the name of the corporation.

Once these four steps are completed, you will have an operational non-profit corporation. However, before the appropriate documents can be prepared, a number of decisions will need to be made. There is no "one size fits all" non-profit corporation. As a result, you will need to tailor the structure of your corporation to fit your particular needs.

Decisions that you need to make

Whether you hire a lawyer experienced in structuring non-profit organizations (especially religious organizations – like me) or decide to walk through the process on your own, there are a few issues that you need to consider and decisions that need to be made before you and/or your lawyer are ready to prepare and file the Articles. The issues that you need to think about include:

What's in a Name?

The first step is the most fun, picking a name for your new corporation. Prior to starting the process, I suggest picking several names (at least 3 or 4) and ranking them in order from favorite to least favorite. Then, you or your lawyer can do a search (on the applicable Secretary of State website) to see if a particular name is available in your State before the documents are prepared and filed. The basic test is whether the name that you want to use is "confusingly similar" with the name already being used by another corporation in your state.

Please note that just because you file organizational documents (usually called the Articles of Organization or the Article of Incorporation, depending on your state) using a particular name, it does not mean that you "own" that name. It only means that no one else in your state can use that name for a corporation. To protect your new corporate name, you will also need to file a trademark application with the federal government and/or state government. While trademark law is beyond the scope of this book, it is worth noting with regard to names, the more unique the better in terms of being able to protect that name. Common names are very difficult to protect. The name of a church or ministry, and the ability to protect it, can be very significant in the modern world. Today, more and more ministries have a significant media presence and sell a significant amount of product through a variety of distribution outlets. As such, these ministries become "brands" that have value. You should talk with your lawyer at the outset about the options for protecting your ministry's name.

Where to Incorporate?

While the decision of where to incorporate a for-profit business can often be a complex process (primarily due to tax and corporate securities law reasons), I simply recommend that you incorporate your church or ministry in the State in which you are based. Since you don't have shareholders and the primary reason to be a non-profit corporation is to become tax-exempt, there is simply not a good reason to go to the extra trouble and expense of an out-of-state incorporation in most cases.

What Happens at the End?

While we all hope and pray that your new church or ministry will be around for hundreds of years, the reality (as I am fond of telling my clients) is that the end will come at some point and you need to think about at the end. Because, as we discussed above, a non-profit corporation is not owned by anyone, the Articles (the organizational document with your State's Secretary of State) are required to include a "dissolution" provision that states what will happen to the assets of the corporation in the event that the corporation is dissolved (closes down). Because non-profit corporations are not owned by anyone, the law requires that all of the corporation's assets be transferred to another non-profit/tax-exempt (later, I will address the distinction between the terms "non-profit" and "tax-exempt") organization in the event of dissolution. You can either specify a particular tax-exempt organization to receive the assets or simply provide that at the time of dissolution, your Board of Directors will select an eligible recipient for the assets. Unless there is a reason to do otherwise, I suggest leaving this decision to the time of dissolution.

The Tax-Exempt Purpose of the Corporation

In order to eligible to be considered "tax-exempt", the Articles need to specify the tax-exempt "purpose" of the corporation for which the corporation was formed. Under the Internal Revenue Code, tax-exempt corporations may be formed for religious, educational, scientific, or charitable purposes. While these are very broad terms, "religious", "charitable", "educational", and "scientific" each have specific meanings under the tax code. If you are forming a corporation that will act as a church or ministry, I suggest that you include religious, charitable and educational as the purposes for the formation of the corporation. Using those three designations will cover practically any activity that a church or ministry may engage in.

For example, "religious" covers all of your basic ministry related activities that are designed to spread the Gospel. "Educational" will cover a school and "charitable" will cover any benevolent activities undertaken by the church, such as food programs.

For tax-exemption purposes, the IRS requires the Articles to include a statement that the corporation "shall be operated exclusively for (insert the purposes such as religious, educational and charitable) purposes as defined by the Internal Revenue Code."

Second, the purpose statements set forth what the corporation was formed to do. I suggest a very broad statement such as "to spread the gospel of Jesus Christ by any means possible." Such a broad statement covers any activity in which a church may engage. The point is to avoid the necessity of having to later re-write of your Articles.

Whether you include a simple statement or prepare something more elaborate, just remember that the document will be public record. Keep in mind that anyone who so desires can go online (in most states) or send a request to the Secretary of State and obtain a copy of your Articles.

What are the Powers of the Corporation?

The Articles also need to specify the "powers" of the corporation – or what types of activities the corporation may engage in. While some lawyers try to list every imaginable thing that a church corporation might do, something inevitably gets left out. Therefore, I simply state that the corporation has all powers available under law. Again, broad, general statements help avoid the need for later revisions.

If your existing corporation has a very specific Powers or Purpose statement, you may want to consider a revision to ensure that all of your current and planned activities are covered.

Whether or Not to Have Members?

Non-profit corporations come in two basic types, those with members and those without members. As a result, the Articles will need to include a statement as to whether or not the Corporation will have members. Then, if the corporation has members, the rights of those members will be set out at some point (usually in the corporation's Bylaws).

Before moving ahead, we need to make an important distinction. While all churches have "members" who join and support the church, you can make a decision as to whether these "members" of the congregation are also "members" for purposes of state corporate law. Under state corporate law, if you choose to have "members" those individuals will have certain rights (similar to shareholders) in the management of the corporation. For example, members are generally entitled to vote on certain issues (like the election of the Board, purchase of property, the sale of the corporation's assets or similar matters). While most states allow non-profit corporations a great deal a latitude to specify (usually in the corporation's Bylaws) exactly what authority the members possess, many states do have statutes that specify certain basic voting rights for members. The important point is that it is possible to have members (for congregational purposes) without granting those members the authority and rights granted to the "members" of non-profit corporations under state corporate law.

That being said, most church organizations will have members and the Bylaws of the church generally provide that the members possess only those rights designated in the Bylaws. The extent of those rights will depend on the type of organizational structure that the particular church chooses.

For a pure ministry (a religious organization that does not operate a church), there is typically no need to have members and a simple statement to that effect is included in the Articles.

Before proceeding, a quick word on the organizational structure of corporations may be beneficial. With a for profit corporation, whether it is General Motors or Al's Burger Barn, there are three layers of power. Ultimate power always resides with the **shareholders** of the corporation. The shareholders own the company and, ultimately call the shots. In turn, the shareholders elect the **Board of Directors** of the Corporation. The Board is the policy and direction setting body of the corporation. Because it is a smaller group, the board meets on a regular basis to oversee the operations of the business. In turn, the Board is charged with electing the **officers** of the corp. The officers are the actual people charged with running the day-to-day operations of the business. The officers include the President. Vice Presidents (if any), Secretary, Treasurer. These people may or may not be board members or shareholders.

With Al's Burger Barn, Al may be the sole shareholder, the Chairman of the Board and the President. Larger companies such as GM delegate power to the board and officers. In a company such as GM that has tens of thousands of shareholders, the board runs the company. However, if enough of the shareholders do not like the way things are being run, they can get together at the annual meeting and replace management.

With a non-profit corporation, the set-up is a little different. There are no owners. A non-profit and its assets do not belong to any individuals. Therefore, there is no preset ultimate authority equivalent to shareholders. However, a non-profit corporation still must rely upon people to run it. Like a for-profit company, a non-profit corporation will have a Board of Directors and officers (with functions similar to their counterparts in a for profit company). A church, unlike a for profit corp., does not have owners and, therefore, has no shareholders. A church, however, typically has members. Those members, while they have no ownership stake, may or may not have a say in how the church is run. It is the organizational documents of the church (the articles and bylaws) that set forth exactly how power is divided among the members, the board and the officers.

In most states, the law grants broad authority for individual non-profit corporations to draft bylaws that match its situation and needs. Therefore, Bylaws can be custom tailored to any given situation. For the most part, however, the organizational structure of churches falls into three broad categories.

First is the traditional congregation driven church. This is the structure used by many southern Baptist churches and other denominational structures. Under this structure, the church congregation is the highest decision making body in the church. The congregation is empowered to vote to make most major decisions and can hire and remove employees of the church up to and including removal of the pastor.

Next is the board driven church. In this type of organization, a relatively small board of directors (sometimes called trustees) has full authority to direct all activities of the church. While the church has members, those members are not granted any actual authority to govern the organization. The members cannot vote to remove a pastor or buy a new building.

The board driven structure can be modified to grant almost complete control to a single individual. For instance, a pastor can be granted perpetual office and the power to remove that pastor can be virtually eliminated. For instance, giving the pastor to right to remove and appoint the other board members gives the pastor unlimited corporate power because he or she can simply replace anyone who is hostile to the pastor.

One word to the wise here, you need to maintain some independence among your board for address topics such as executive compensation. The point is that ultimately you need your lawyer to prepare balanced Bylaws to look to the big picture and do not get obsessed with preventing an overthrow. The pastor's real authority is moral, not legal authority.

Third model is the hybrid structure. With a hybrid church, the members retain ultimate power on a few specific issues. For example, it is common for a hybrid structure church to have members that vote only to (i) elect a board of directors of the church who govern the day-to-day operations, (ii) remove and/or hire a pastor (usually requires a super majority of 75-80%, (iii) take on indebtedness to purchase property, or (iv) amend the Bylaws. You can see that in such a structure, the board and staff have the authority to run day-to-day operations, but the members retain the ultimate controls. Most important of the powers is the power to amend the Bylaws. The power to amend the Bylaws is the power to change the rules when it suits you.

Before moving on, a couple of quick points should be made about Bylaws. First, under most state laws, any officer, director or member of a non-profit corporation is entitled to inspect its books and records. This means that most church members have the right to see all of the books and records of your church. However, if your structure places no power in the hands of your members, you can avoid this issue by providing, in your Bylaws, that the members of your church are not members of the corporation for the purposes of state law and those church members have none of the powers granted to members under state law.

Next, please note that the sample Bylaws provides that the corporation may not make a loan to its officers or directors. This section is included because it reflects the law of most states. Generally, all board members who approve such a loan are liable for its repayment until the debtor does in fact repay the loan.

The Registered Agent

The Articles will need list the name and street address (post office boxes are not allowed) of the person or entity (the registered agent can be another corporation or LLC) who will serve as the registered agent of the corporation. This person will serve two primary functions. First, this individual will be the addressee of any official mail from the state. Therefore, the name and address must be good because the state will assume that any mailed documents were in fact received. Second, this person will most likely be the person who is served with any lawsuit that is filed against the church. Therefore, use a trustworthy individual and an address that is not likely to change often (the address of the church is usually better than the address of an individual). When the person or address changes, you simply need to file a change form with the Secretary of State and pay a small fee.

This simple issue creates more problems for churches that almost any other corporate matter. Most states will periodically send out "public information" forms to all corporations. The forms are mailed to the registered agent at the registered address and are required to be completed and returned within a specified time period. If the form is not returned, the corporation will be forfeited. This means that the corporation will cease to exist as a legal entity. This happens all the time. Worse, it is always discovered at a critical time – usually when the lawsuit has arrived and the pastor is being sued personally because no corporation exists or just before you are about to close on a building loan.

The point is a simple one. Someone needs to make sure this information stays up to date.

The Board of Directors

All non-profit corporations are required to have a board of

directors. Just as with for profit companies the board is responsible for running the corporation and making major decisions. Accordingly, the board members should be people that you trust and respect. In addition, board members should be able to add value to the organization.

In most states, you are required to name a minimum of three (3) board members and you can have as many directors as you like. However, to avoid the potential for stalemates, you should avoid having an even number of people on the board (a four person board can be divided two against two). In addition, large boards become cumbersome (it can be difficult to set-up meetings) and hard to manage (increasing the board size increases the potential for having board members with different personal agendas etc). I suggest creating a board of three or five members at the outset.

As will be discussed later, the board is either the most powerful entity in your corporate structure or the second most powerful. In some cases, the church membership is empowered to elect the board members and, as a result, the membership retains ultimate power under such a structure. In other cases, the corporation is structured so that the board elects itself or is appointed by an individual or committee. In these cases, the board is the most powerful entity in the corporation.

Choosing a good board is vital to the long-term success of your corporation. A board of yes men will provide no real assistance or guidance. On the other hand, a renegade board can cause division. You need smart, serious people who can add value to your ministry.

Prior to concluding this section, a quick word on the duty and obligation of board members is in order. Very often, potential board members have a concern for their personal liability. As a result, they decline to serve and the church is denied the benefit of their knowledge because they fear the unknown. In a properly structured corporation, board members have very little to fear. As long as the corporation organizational documents provide for limitation of officer's and director's liability as well as indemnification (as discussed below), the individual officers and directors will be protected from most liability for any official act taken in the course of their corporate duties.

As a general matter, the only time an officer or director will not be covered is rare occasion when a corporation cannot offer protection. This occurs when an officer or director has violated his or her duty of loyalty and good faith to the corporation. A director has a duty to act in good faith in a manner that the director reasonably believes to be in the best interest of the corporation. This basically means that the director has a duty to try and to do what he or she believes is best for the corporation. This does not mean that the director has to make the right decisions all the time (no one can). It only means that the director has to try to make the right decisions.

The most common example of a director violating this duty of loyalty and good faith is when a director engages in undisclosed self-dealing. Generally, there is no prohibition against a member of your board of directors engaging in a business transaction with your church (subject to certain IRS restrictions which are discussed in my Wallace Church Law Series e-book *How to Get and Protect Your Ministry's Tax-Exempt Status*). However, two simple rules need to be met. First, the board members interest in the transaction should be disclosed to the full board and approved by a majority of the other board members (the involved board member should not vote on the item). Secondly, the transaction should be fair to the corporation.

Here is an example. Your church is looking for land to build a new sanctuary. Elder Joe, a board member, is in the real estate business and suggests that the board look at a tract land that he has seen. Elder Joe does not disclose that he owns the company that owns the land. He then tells the board that the land is a great deal and that the church should sign the purchase contract. If it turns out that the land is worth half of what Elder Joe said and he never disclosed his interest in the deal, Joe has violated his duty of good faith and loyalty to the church. Because Elder Joe put his personal best interest above the best interest of the church, he violated his duty of loyalty to the church and he may face liability as a result.

Another example of violating your duty of good faith is by following a course of action that you know is wrong and continuing despite your knowledge that the act is wrong or illegal. It is clearly a violation of this duty to engage in conduct you know is wrong.

One final note, board members need to make an effort to be right. This means attending meetings on a regular basis, gathering information and making a decision. Generally, board members are protected if they rely on information provided by officers of the corporation and the corporation's attorneys and accountants, unless you have reason to know that the information provided is false or if you now the person providing the information is unqualified to do so. As long as the information appears to be credible and from a credible source, board members may rely upon the data in making decisions.

Similar rules apply to the officers of the church. Like board members they have a duty of good faith and loyalty to the corporation. As a result, they also have a duty to try to do the right thing. The bottom line is that as long as you reasonably believe that the action you are taking is in the best interest of the corporation, you will find protection under today's corporate laws.

The No-No's

Either the Articles or bylaws (discussed later) also should include a statement of activities that the corporation will not engage in. This restrictions are designed to insure that you will operate your church or ministry in compliance with the essence of the regulations that govern non-profit corporations. Basically, these rules all come down to the fact that you need to operate your ministry for its exempt purposes and not for the benefit of any individual.

However, the restrictions go back to the concept that individuals do not own a non-profit corporation. The public at large is the beneficiary of the corporation's assets. Therefore, you need to keep in mind that the best interest of the organization should be placed ahead of the best interest of the individuals who operate the ministry or church. As a result, any dealings between a non-profit corporation and those people who control it must be fair and arms-length.

One important restriction relates to what political activities a church or ministry may participate in. The IRS rules do not prohibit all political activities. However, you do need to follow this simple rule of thumb – It is ok to encourage your congregation to be politically active (telling the church members to be sure to vote next Tuesday in the election); and it is ok to teach whether a particular act is right or wrong (telling the church your views on an issue such as abortion); but it is not ok to tell your church who to vote for and it is not ok for the church to expend its funds on political causes or candidates. In other words, you can support issues and activism, but not individual candidates.

Remember, you, as an individual, are separate from the church as an entity. Therefore, the pastor can give his or her personal money to a candidate. A minister can support or endorse a candidate – they just should not do it from the pulpit.

If you are going to permit political candidates to visit your church, I suggest that you invite the candidates from both parties. In addition, there is no problem with inviting office holders to special events, such as dedications or anniversaries. An invitation or an appearance by a political office holder is not an endorsement. Just keep the issues separate.

That being said, I encourage all church leaders to take the time to get to know and develop relationships with governmental leaders at all levels. Any large church will find itself frequently doing business with the government, especially local city and county officials. When doing so, there is no substitute for relationships.

When it comes to dealing with the government, churches generally operate at a significant disadvantage. Governments need tax revenue to operate and churches do not pay taxes. This simple fact means that churches, from a financial standpoint, are liabilities, not assets, to a city government. Therefore, some cities can be less than accommodating to churches. The best way to overcome this setback is to develop relationships. This takes time and effort, but it always pays off.

Limitation of Liability for Officers and Directors

As a ministry leader, it is also important that your Articles or Bylaws include statements limiting the liability of officers and directors to the greatest extent possible. Most states allow a corporation to agree, in its Articles or Bylaws, to relieve its board members and officers of liability to the corporation for any acts, unless those acts violate the board members duties of loyalty and good faith and fair dealing to the corporation.

Because of this, all board members need to understand these

concepts. Boiled down, a board member has an obligation to act in good faith to do what is best for the corporation. The board member cannot put his or her own interest above that of the corporation. It also means that the board member has an obligation to TRY to do the right thing. There is no obligation that the board member be right 100% of the time, only an obligation to try.

In the real world this means that the board member needs to regularly attend meetings, attempt to be informed about the decisions that are being made and not act out of self-interest.

Here is a quick example of how this works. Deacon Wilson is one of your board members and is in the real estate business. The church needs property for a new building and Deacon Wilson is in charge of the search. Deacon Wilson has a duty to find the best deal for the church. But if Deacon Wilson reports back that certain a property is the only one that works and it available for only $1,000,000; but fails to tell the rest of the board that he owns that property, that it is only worth $500,000 and that 5 other cheaper and better properties exist. Then, in that case, Deacon Wilson has violated his duty of loyalty and good faith to the corporation and the corporation can sue him if they acted on his information.

It is worth noting that if Deacon Wilson's property really is the best choice, it is ok for the church to buy it as long as the deal is fair and he discloses his interest and does not vote on the decision. Remember that Deacon Wilson cannot use the corporation for his own self-interest or benefit.

Indemnification of Officers and Directors

Well-drafted Articles and/or Bylaws will also contain a provision providing that the Corporation will indemnify its officers and directors for actions taken in the course of their official duties, to the greatest extent allowed by law. This provision provides critical protection for the individuals who run the church. Very often when a church, as a corporation, is sued for some alleged misconduct (for instance, a former employee sues alleging sexual harassment), the individual board members of the church may also sued (usually based on some idea that the individual allowed the wrong to occur). When that happens, you, as an individual who has been sued, will need to obtain counsel to defend you and your interests (your interests may or may not differ from the interests of the church) and that will cost money. If the Articles (or Bylaws) have been drafted properly, you will be able to look to the church for protection.

By agreeing in the Articles (or Bylaws) to indemnify its officers and directors, the church is saying that it will defend you in case you are sued as a result of your official acts. This means the church will hire a lawyer to represent you and also pay any judgment if you lose that lawsuit.

In addition, this indemnity will not extend to acts that violate the duty of good faith or loyalty. At the point in time that the corporation determines that the director in question violated his duty to the corporation the corporation may drop its defense.

One important note here, just because a church has agreed in the Articles or Bylaws to indemnify it officers and directors, it does not guarantee that the church will have the capacity to follow-through on that promise. Accordingly, you need to insist that your church obtain Directors and Officers insurance as part of its standard insurance package. This coverage will provide the funding to allow the church to meet its commitments in the event that its officer or directors are sued.

BYLAWS

At the same time the Articles are prepared, you or your lawyer will need to prepare Bylaws for the corporation. Together with the Articles, the Bylaws form the governing documents of the corporation. In essence, the Bylaws set forth the rules for operating the corporation. As I always tell my clients, the Bylaws are largely meaningless until there is a dispute about some course of action the church is going to take (such as a decision to remove a Board member or Pastor, or make some other major decision),then the Bylaws become all important. As the corporate rulebook, the Bylaws will set forth all of the formal rules that a corporation needs to follow to implement an official course of action.

As a pastor or board member, you need to review your Bylaws and understand the rules that apply in the event of a dispute. For example, what if there were to be a split in your church. If two groups want to move in disparate directions, the Bylaws will inevitably dictate who will wins the battle and the war. The Bylaws accomplish this by setting out who has the power to take a specific action.

For example, I know of a church split that occurred between a young pastor and a board controlled by the allies of the recently retired pastor and church founder. As sometimes happens, the retired pastor was not really ready to let go and he used his allies on the board to drive out the new young pastor. Despite the ability and popularity of the young pastor, this war was over before it ever started because the Articles and Bylaws of the church gave the small board ultimate authority over the pastor and the will of the congregation. The young pastor's only option was to leave and start a new church. If you take over a situation, learn what the ground rules are. Without this knowledge, you are unprepared to act.

ORGANIZATIONAL MEETING

After Articles have been drafted and filed and the Bylaws have been prepared, the third step in the organizational process to hold an organizational meeting of the board of directors. The board members name in the Articles need have their first meeting to take care of a few housekeeping matters. Very often, this first meeting is done by written consent (all of the named directors sign a consent resolution). At this meeting, the following actions need to be taken:

1.   The Articles and the Bylaw need to be approved and ratified.
2.   A Minute Book for keeping the Articles, Bylaws and Minutes need to be approved.
3.   The Board needs to elect the initial officers of the corporation. Most states require the corporation to elect at least a President and a Secretary. As a general matter, the President is charged with running the corporation. The Senior Pastor is typically named the President of the corporation. The Secretary is charged with maintaining corporate records. For a   more detailed description of duties, see the sample Bylaws in the Appendix.

A couple of quick points should be made about the Organizational Meeting. With regard to board membership, it is common for the board members of churches to serve without compensation. This is often a good idea and offers a distinct benefit. By serving without pay, board members are designated as "volunteers" and are afforded greater latitude by the courts. By this I mean that a court will not expect a volunteer board members to exercise as much diligence as a paid board member. In addition, some states offer limited legal protections for volunteers serving non-profit organizations.

The next step to forming your non-profit corporation's to apply for and receive your corporation's **Employer Identification Number (EIN) (also referred to as a Tax ID Number)**. This number is the equivalent of a social security number for a corporation. It is required to open a corporate bank account or conduct similar official business in the name of the corporation. Obtaining the number is a simple process. You simply or go online to www.irs.gov and provide the IRS with the information requested (it takes about 5 minutes) and they will assign the number to you immediately and then send a confirmation letter.

The last step is to set-up bank accounts for the corporation. Your bank will need a copy of the Articles (with the evidence of filing provided by your state), a copy of the signed Bylaws and your EIN.

At this point, you now have an official non-profit corporation. While this may appear to be time consuming and complex, it is really a simple process and can be completed literally within a day or two. The key is to have an understanding of the type of organizational structure that you want to have in place. If you are not sure, that is fine too. You can always amend your Articles of Incorporation or Bylaws to implement a new structure (as long as all of the required parties agree).

Multiple Corporations

Sometimes, it is advisable for a church or ministry to form multiple corporations because of the nature of their activities. Basically, the time and expense of forming additional corporations is worth it in two cases. First, when a church engages in high-risk activities, consideration should be given to isolating these activities in a stand-alone corporation. The purpose of this would be to protect the assets of the main church corporation in the event that the corporation housing the high-risk activities is sued and found liable for damages in an amount greater than the available insurance.

A common example is a school. Because schools involve the oversight of large numbers of young children, there is always the chance of liability. What happens if a teacher, for example, sexually assaults a student and the school is found liable for $10,000,000 in damages but only has $5,000,000 in available insurance. If a stand-alone corporation operates the school, only the assets of that corporation are subject to being seized to pay the judgment. However, if the church operates the school through the same corporation as the church, then the assets of the church are subject to the judgment.

One note here, in some states non-profit corporations are given special protections from many types of lawsuits. If you are in one of those states, such as Texas, your lawyer can take those available protections into account when trying to help you evaluate the risk level of your activities and whether a separate corporation is needed.

The other time a separate corporation is needed is when you want to engage in activities that would create liability for unrelated business income taxes. For instance, real estate investments by the church or other investments in businesses may create unrelated business income. In those cases, it is wise to isolate that income (and the need to pay taxes) in a corporation separate from the church. This will prevent the church from having to file a tax return (and consequently disclosing private financial information).

Conclusion

I hope that this e-book has been helpful to you and your ministry. If you are looking for help on other church law matters, look for the other e-books in the Wallace Church Law Series.

If I can be of service to you or your ministry, please do not hesitate to contact me at curtis@curtiswallace.net.

The following pages contain an Appendix with sample documents, including a Certificate of Formation, Bylaws, Organizational Consent and a Conflicts of Interest Policy.

APPENDIX

Certificate of Formation
<u>Non-Profit Corporation</u>

Article 1 – Corporate Name

The filing entity formed is a non-profit corporation. The name of the entity is "Wallace Ministries, Inc."

Article 2 – Registered Agent and Registered Office

The initial registered agent is _____________________, an individual residing in the State of Texas. The business address of the registered agent and the registered office address is ____________________. The consent of the registered agent is maintained by the corporation.

Article 3 – Organizational Structure

The corporation shall not have members.

Article 4 – Management

The management of the affairs of the corporation shall be vested in its board of directors. The initial board of directors shall consist of three (3) members. The names and addresses of the initial board members are as follows:

____

____

____

Article 5 – Purpose and Powers

The corporation is organized and its assets shall be used solely and exclusively for educational, religious and educational purposes, as defined by Section 501(c)(3) of the Internal Revenue Code, as amended.

The corporation shall have the power to engage in any lawful activity for which non-profit corporations may be incorporated in the State of Texas.

Article 6 – Dissolution

Upon the dissolution of the corporation, its assets shall be distributed to another organization selected by the Board of Directors that qualifies as a tax-exempt organization pursuant to Section 501(c)(3) of the Internal Revenue Code, as amended.

Article 7 – Effectiveness of Filing

This document becomes effective upon its filing with the Texas Secretary of State.

Article 8 - Organizer

The name and address of the organizer of the corporation are as follows:

Curtis W. Wallace
1527 West State Highway 114
Suite 500
Grapevine, Texas 76051

The undersigned affirms that the person designated as registered agent has consented to the appointment. The undersigned signs this document subject to the penalties imposed by law for submission of a materially false or fraudulent instrument and certifies under penalty of perjury that the undersigned is authorized under the provisions of law governing the entity to execute the filing instrument.

____

Curtis W. Wallace, Organizer

BYLAWS
OF
WALLACE MINISTRIES, INC.

These Bylaws (the "Bylaws") govern the affairs of Wallace Ministries, Inc. (the "Ministry"), organized under Texas Non-Profit Corporation Act, as amended (the "Act").

1. OFFICES

1.01	The principal office of the Ministry shall be located at [INSERT ADDRESS] or such other location may be determined by the Board of Directors, from time to time.

1.02	The Ministry shall comply with the Act and maintain a registered office and registered agent in Texas. The registered office may, but need not, be identical with the Ministry's principal office. The Board of Directors may change the registered office and/or registered agent as provided in the Act.

2. STATEMENT OF FAITH

[PLEASE NOTE THAT I SUGGEST THE INCLUSION OF A STATEMENT OF FAITH IN THE BYLAWS FOR ALL RELIGIOUS NON-PROFITS. CHURCHES AND MINISTRIES HAVE CONSTITUTIONAL PROTECTIONS AVAILABLE TO THEM FOR ACTIONS TAKEN IN ACCORDANCE WITH THEIR HONESTLY

2.01   The Bible (2 Timothy 3:16-17; 2 Peter 1:20-21; Hebrews 4:12)
We believe that the Scriptures in all 66 books of the Old and New Testaments
are verbally inspired of God, error free in the original manuscripts, and the
supreme authority of faith and practice for followers of Christ.

2.02   God (Deuteronomy 6:4)
We believe there is one living and true God, who is one in essence, while
eternally existing in three distinct persons; Father, Son and Holy Spirit.

2.03   Man (Genesis 1:26-27; Romans 1:18-32, 3:10-23)
We believe that mankind was directly created in the image of God to enjoy
His fellowship and fulfill His purposes on earth. However, in Adam, all
mankind fell into sin; consequently all people are spiritually dead and subject
to the certainty of both physical and spiritual death apart from faith in Jesus
Christ.

2.04   Salvation (John 1:12, 3:16, 14:6; Ephesians 2:8-9)
We believe that salvation is by grace, through faith in Jesus Christ. All who
believe in Him are declared righteous by the Father on the grounds of Jesus
Christ's life, death and resurrection, being regenerated by and baptized in the
Holy Spirit.

2.05   The Church (Acts 2:41-47; Hebrews 10:24-25; 1 Corinthians
12-14)
We believe that all who are "born again" by the Holy Spirit belong to the one
true church and are instructed by the Scriptures to associate themselves in
local, visible churches.

2.06   Ordinances (Matt. 28:18-20; Romans 6:3-7; 1 Corinthians
11:23-29)
Baptism is a clear injunction of the Scriptures which outwardly expresses the
inward reality of new life in Christ. Our method of baptism is immersion as
described in the New Testament and practiced in the early church.

2.07   We believe that the Lord's Supper is a memorial of Christ and

His redemptive death. It is also an expression of our fellowship with one another. In communion we are reminded of Christ's first coming and encouraged to look forward to His coming again.

2.08		The Future (Matthew 24-25; 1 Thessalonians 4:13-18)
We believe the next great event of human history will be the personal return of Jesus Christ. This is the blessed hope for which all those who love Christ yearn. While the exact time of Christ's return is unknown, it is imminent and certain.

3. MEMBERS

3.01		The Ministry shall not have members.

[IF YOUR CORPORATION WILL HAVE MEMBERS, YOU WILL INCLUDE PROVISIONS HERE SPECIFYING THE RIGHTS AND OBLIGATIONS OF THE MEMBERS AS WELL AS THE CRITERIA FOR MEMBERSHIP]

4. BOARD OF DIRECTORS

4.01		The affairs of the Ministry shall be managed by the Board of Directors.

4.02		The number of Directors shall be determined by the Board of Directors, but such number shall not be less than three (3), nor greater than nine (9). The initial Board of Directors shall consist of five (5) members. Each Director shall serve for a term of one (1) year. There is no limit on the number of terms that a Director may serve.

4.03		Directors shall be elected, annually, by the Board of Directors.

4.04		Any vacancy occurring in the Board of Directors, and any position to be filled as a result of an increase in the number of Directors, shall be filled by a vote of the Board of Directors. A Director appointed to fill a vacancy shall be appointed for the remainder of the term of the predecessor on office. There is no limit on the number of terms that a Director may serve.

4.05		The annual meeting of the Board of Directors shall take place at a date and time specified by the Board of Directors.

4.06	The Board of Directors may provide for regular meetings by a resolution setting forth the time and place for such meetings. The meetings shall be held at the principal office of the Ministry, unless the resolution states otherwise. No notice of the regular meetings, other than the resolution establishing the same, shall be required.

4.07	Special Meetings of the Board of Directors may be called by or at the request of the President or any two (2) Directors. The person (s) requesting the meeting shall notify the Secretary of the Ministry who shall send a notice specifying the time and place for the special meeting of the Board of Directors, in accordance with the Bylaws.

4.08	Written notice of any special meeting of the Board of Directors shall be delivered to each Director not less than three (3) nor more than thirty (30) days before the date of the meeting. The notice shall state the time, place, and date of meeting, who called the meeting and the purpose(s) for which the meeting was called.

4.09	A majority of the number of Directors then in office shall constitute a quorum for the transaction of business at any meeting of the Board of Directors. The Directors present at a duly called meeting at which a quorum is present may continue to transact business even if a sufficient number of Directors leave the meeting so that a quorum is no longer present. However, no action may be approved without the vote of at least a majority of the number of Directors required to make a quorum. If a quorum is not present at any time during a meeting, the majority of those present may adjourn and reconvene the meeting one time without further notice.

4.10	The Board of Directors may meet by telephone conference or video conference.

4.11	Any action that may be taken at a meeting of the Board of Directors may be taken by unanimous written consent of all members of the Board of Directors.

4.12	A Director may vote by written proxy executed by the Director pursuant to of these Bylaws.

4.13	Directors shall discharge their duties, including any duties as committee members in good faith, with ordinary care and in a manner they reasonably believe to be in the best interest of the Ministry. In the discharge of any duty imposed or power conferred on Directors, they may, in good faith, rely on information, opinions, reports or statement, including financial statements and other financial data, concerning the Ministry or another person that were prepared or presented by a variety of persons, including officers and employees of the Ministry, professional advisors or experts such as lawyers, accountants and consultants. A Director is not acting in good faith if the Director has knowledge concerning a matter in question that renders reliance unwarranted.

4.14   Directors are not deemed to have the duties of a trustee of a trust with respect to the Ministry or property held by the Ministry, including property that may be subject to restrictions imposed by the donor of the property.

4.15   Directors are entitled to select advisors and delegate duties and responsibilities to them; such as power to acquire stocks, bonds, securities and other investments on behalf of the Ministry. The Directors have no liability for actions taken or omitted by the advisor of the Director acts in good faith and with ordinary acre in selecting the advisor.

4.16   Contracts or transactions between the Ministry and Directors or officers who have a financial interest in the matter are not void or voidable solely for that reason. Nor is the contract or transaction void or voidable solely because the Director or Officer is present at or participates in the meeting that authorizes the contract or transaction, or solely because the interested party's vote is counted for the purpose. However, the material facts must be disclosed to the Board of Directors, the transaction must be fair to the Ministry and a majority of disinterested Directors present at the meeting must have approved of the contract or transaction.

4.17   The Board of Directors shall try to act by consensus. However, a vote of a majority of Directors present at a duly called meeting (if notice is required) at which a quorum is present shall be sufficient to constitute an act of the Board of Directors, unless a greater number is required by the Bylaws or the Act.

4.18   Unless the Board of Directors determines otherwise, the Directors shall serve without salaries. The Board of Directors may adopt a resolution providing that the Ministry reimburse Directors for the cost of attending meetings. A Director may serve the Ministry in another capacity and receive reasonable compensation for those services.

4.19   At any time, any Director may be removed from the Board of Directors by a two-thirds vote of the Board of Directors.

5. OFFICERS

5.01   The officers of the Ministry shall include a president, a secretary, and a treasurer (the secretary and treasurer may be the same person) and may include any number of vice presidents, assistant secretary, assistant treasurer or other officer positions created and defined by the Board of Directors. Any two or more offices may be held by the same person, subject to the requirements of the Act.

5.02   The President shall be the chief executive officer of the Ministry. The President shall supervise and control all of the day to day business and affairs of the Ministry, subject to the direction of the Board of Directors. The President shall preside at all meetings of the Board of Directors (if he is in attendance). The President may execute any deeds, mortgages, bonds, contracts or other instruments that the Board of Directors has authorized to be executed.

5.03   When the President is absent, is unable to act or refuses to act, a Vice President shall perform the duties of the President; subject to the directions or limitations put in place by the Board of Directors. A Vice President shall perform such other duties as assigned by the President or the Board of Directors. Unless authorized by the Board of Directors, a Vice President shall not have authority to sign contracts or otherwise bind the Ministry.

5.04   The Treasurer shall:
        (a) have charge and custody of, and be responsible for, all funds and securities of the Ministry;
        (b) receive and give receipts for moneys due and payable to the Ministry from any source;
        (c) deposit all monies of the Ministry in the name of the Ministry in banks, trust companies or other depositories as directed by the Board of

Directors;

(d) write checks and disburse funds to pay the obligations of the Ministry;

(e) maintain the financial books and records of the Ministry;

(f) prepare regular financial statements for the Ministry;

(g) perform other duties as assigned by the President or the Board of Directors of the Ministry;

(h) if required by the Board of Directors, give a bond for the faithful discharge of his or her duties in a sum and with a surety determined by the Board of Directors (such bond shall be at the sole cost of the Ministry);

(i) perform all other duties incident to the office of treasurer.

5.05   The Secretary shall:

(a) give all notices as provided in the Bylaws or as required by the Act.

(b) take minutes of the meetings of the Board of Directors and maintain such minutes as part of the records of the Ministry;

(c) maintain custody of the corporate records and the seal, if any, of the Ministry;

(d) affix the seal of the Ministry to all documents as authorized and required;

(e) keep a register of the address and other contact information of each director, officer and employee of the Ministry;

(f) perform such other duties as assigned by the President or Board oF Directors;

(g) perform all other duties incident to the office of Secretary.

5.06   The officers of the Ministry shall be elected annually by the Board of Directors. Each officer shall hold office until a successor is duly elected and qualified; unless such officer is deceased or has been removed by the Board of Directors in which case the officer's term in office will have automatically ended on the death or removal from office of such officer.

5.07   Any officer may be removed by the Board of Directors, with or without good cause. The removal of any officer shall be without prejudice to the contract rights, if any, of the officer.

5.08   Any vacancy in any office shall be filled by the Board of

Directors for the remainder of the unexpired term of the office.

6. COMMITTEES

6.01   The Board of Directors may adopt a resolution establishing one or more committees, delegating specified authority to a committee, and appointing or removing members of a committee. A committee shall include one or more Directors and may include persons who are not Directors. If the committee includes one or more persons who are not Directors, the committee may not exercise any authority reserved to the Board of Directors under the Bylaws or the Act. No committee shall have the authority of the Board of Directors to:

> (a) Amend the Articles of Incorporation or Bylaws of the Ministry;
> (b) Adopt a plan of merger or consolidation with another entity;
> (c) Authorize the sale, lease, exchange or mortgage of all or substantially all of the Ministry's assets;
> (d) Authorize the dissolution of the Ministry;
> (e) Revoke proceedings for the dissolution of the Ministry;
> (f) Adopt a plan for distribution of the Ministry's assets
> (g) Elect, appoint or remove a member of a committee;
> (h) Approve any transaction that involves a potential conflict of interest;
> (i) Take any action outside of the scope of authority delegated to it by the Board of Directors

6.02   Each member of a committee shall continue to serve on the committee until the next annual meeting of the members of the Ministry and until a successor is appointed. However, the term of a committee member may terminate earlier if the committee is terminated or if the member dies, ceases to qualify, resigns, or is removed as a member. A vacancy on a committee may be filled by an appointment made in the same manner as an original appointment. A person appointed to fill a vacancy shall serve for the remainder of the portion of the terminated committee member's term.

6.03   One member of each committee shall be designated as the chair of the committee and another member of each committee shall be designated as the vice-chair. The chair and the vice-chair shall be elected by the member

of the committee. The chair shall call and preside at all the meetings of the
committee. When the chair is absent, is unable to act, or refuses to act, the
vice-chair shall perform the duties of the chair. When a vice-chair acts in
place of the chair, the vice-chair shall have all the powers of and be subject to
all the restrictions upon the chair.

6.04   Written on printed notice of a committee meeting shall be
delivered to each member of a committee not less than seven (7) nor more
than thirty (30) days before the date of the meeting. The notice shall state the
place, day, and time of the meeting, and the purpose or purposes for which
the meeting is called.

6.05   One half the number of members of a committee shall constitute
a quorum for the transaction of business at any meeting of the committee.
The committee members present at a duly called or held meeting at which a
quorum is present may continue to transact business even if enough
committee members leave the meeting so that less than a quorum remains.
However, no action may be approved without the vote of at least a majority
of the number of committee members require to constitute a quorum. If a
quorum is present at no time during a meeting, the chair may adjourn and
reconvene the meeting one time without further notice.

6.06   Committees shall try to take action by consensus. However, the
vote of a majority of committee members present and voting at a meeting at
which a quorum is present shall be sufficient to constitute the act of the
committee unless the act of a greater number is required by law or the
bylaws. A committee member who is present at a meeting and abstains from
a vote is considered to be present and voting for the purpose of determining
the act of the committee.

6.07   A committee member may vote by proxy executed in writing by
the committee member. No proxy shall be valid after three months from the
date of its execution.

6.08   Committee members shall not receive salaries for their services.
The Board of Directors may adopt a resolution providing for payment to
committee members of the expenses of attendance, if any, for attendance at
each meeting of the committee. A committee member may serve the
Ministry in any other capacity and receive compensation for those services.

Any compensation that the Ministry pays to a committee member shall be commensurate with the services performed and shall be reasonable in amount.

6.09   Each committee may adopt rules for its own operation not inconsistent with the bylaws or with rules adopted by the Board of Directors.

7. TRANSACTIONS OF THE MINISTRY

7.01   The Board of Directors may authorize any officer or agent of the Ministry to enter into a contract or execute and deliver any instrument in the name of and on behalf of the Ministry. This authority may be limited to a specific contract or instrument or it may extend to any number and type of possible contracts and instruments.

7.02   All funds of the Ministry shall be deposited to the credit of the Ministry in banks, trust companies, or other depositaries that the Board of Directors selects.

7.03   The Board of Directors may accept on behalf of the Ministry any contribution, gift, bequest, or devise for the general purposes or for any special of the Ministry. The Board of Directors may make gifts and give charitable contributions that are not prohibited by these Bylaws, the Articles of Incorporation, state law, and requirements for maintaining the Ministry's federal and state tax exempt status.

7.04   The Ministry shall not make any loan to a director or officer of the Ministry. A director, officer, or committee member of the Ministry may lend money to and otherwise transact business with the Ministry except as otherwise provided by the Bylaws, Articles of Incorporation, and all applicable laws. Such a person transacting business with the Ministry has the same rights and obligations relating to those matters as other persons transacting business with the Ministry. The Ministry shall not borrow money from or otherwise transact business with a director, officer, or committee member of the Ministry unless the transaction is described fully in a legally binding instrument and is in the best interest of the Ministry. The Ministry shall not borrow money from or otherwise transact business with a director, officer, or committee member of the Ministry without full disclosure of all relevant facts and without the approval of the Board of Directors, not including the vote of any person having a personal interest in the transaction.

7.05   As long as the Ministry is in existence, and except with the prior approval of the Board of Directors, no director, officer, or committee member of the Ministry shall:

> (a) Do any act in violation of the Bylaws.
> (b) Do any act with the intention of harming the Ministry or any of its operations.
> (c) Do any act that would make it impossible or unnecessarily difficult to carry on the intended or ordinary business of the Ministry.
> (d) Receive an improper personal benefit from the operation of the Ministry.
> (e) Use the assets of this Ministry, directly or indirectly, for any purpose other than carrying on the business of this Ministry.
> (f) Wrongfully transfer or dispose of Ministry property, including intangible property such as good will.
> (g) Use the name of the Ministry (or any substantially similar name) or any trademark or trade name adopted by the Ministry, except on behalf of the Ministry in the ordinary course of the Ministry's business.
> (h) Disclose any of the Ministry business practices, trade secrets, or any other information not generally known to the business community to any person not authorized to receive it.

8. BOOKS AND RECORDS

8.01   The Ministry shall keep correct and complete books and records of account. The Ministry's books and records shall include:

> (a) A file-endorsed copy of all documents filed with the Texas Secretary of State relating to the Ministry, including, but not limited to, the Charter, and any articles of amendment, restated articles, articles of merger, articles of consolidation, and statement of change of registered office or registered agent.

> (b) A copy of the bylaws, and any amended versions or amendments to the bylaws.

> (c) Minutes of the proceedings of the Board of Directors, and committees having any of the authority of the Board of Directors.

(d) A list of the names and addresses of the directors, officers, and any committee members of the Ministry.

(e) If prepared, a financial statement showing the assets, liabilities, and net worth of the Ministry at the end of the three most recent fiscal years.

(f) If prepared, a financial statement showing the income and expenses of the Ministry for the three most recent fiscal years.

(g) All rulings, letters, and other documents relating to the Ministry's federal, state, and local tax status.

8.02   Any director may inspect and receive copies of all books and records of the Ministry required to be kept by the Bylaws. Such a person may inspect or receive copies if the person has a proper purpose related to the person's interest in the Ministry and if the person submits a request in writing. Any person entitled to inspect and copy the Ministry's books and records may do so through his or her attorney or other duly authorized representative. A person entitled to inspect the Ministry's books and records may do so at a reasonable time no later than five working days after the Ministry's receipt of a proper written request. The Board of Directors may establish reasonable fees for copying the Ministry's books and records by members. The fees may cover the cost of materials and labor, but may not exceed fifty cents per page. The Ministry shall provide requested copies of books or records no later than five working days after the Ministry's receipt of a proper written request.

9. FISCAL YEAR

The fiscal year of the Ministry shall begin on the first day of January and end on the last day in December in each year.

10. INDEMNIFICATION

10.01   To the greatest extent permitted by the Act, the Ministry shall indemnify any director, officer, committee member, employee, or agent of the Ministry who was, is, or may be named defendant or respondent in any proceeding as a result of his or her actions or omissions within the scope of his or her official capacity in the Ministry.

10.02(a) Before the Ministry may pay any indemnification expenses (including attorney's fees), the Ministry shall specifically determine that indemnification is permissible, authorize indemnification, and determine that expenses be reimbursed are reasonable. The Ministry may make these determinations and decisions by any one of the following procedures:

  (i) Majority vote of a quorum consisting of directors who, at the time of the vote, are not named defendants or respondents in the proceeding.

  (ii) If such a quorum cannot be obtained, by a majority vote of a committee of the Board of Directors, designated to act in the matter by a majority vote of all directors, consisting solely of two or more directors who at the time of the vote are not named defendants or respondents in the proceeding.

  (iii) Determination by special legal counsel selected by the Board of Directors by vote as provided herein, or if such a quorum cannot be obtained and such a committee cannot be established, by a majority vote of all directors.

  (b) The Ministry shall authorize indemnification and determine that expenses to be reimbursed are reasonable in the same manner that it determines whether indemnification is permissible. If the determination that indemnification is permissible is made by special legal counsel, authorization of indemnification and determination of reasonableness of expenses shall be made in the manner specified herein, governing the selection of special legal counsel. A provision contained in the Articles of Incorporation, these Bylaws, or a resolution of members or the Board of Directors that requires the indemnification permitted by paragraph 10.01 above, constitutes sufficient authorization of indemnification even though the provision may not have been adopted or authorized in the same manner as the determination that indemnification is permissible.

  (c) The Ministry shall pay indemnification expenses before final disposition of a proceeding only after the Ministry determines that the facts then known would not preclude indemnification and the Ministry receives a written affirmation and undertaking from the person to be indemnified. The determination that the facts then known to those making the determination would not preclude indemnification and authorization of payment shall be made in the same manner as a determination that indemnification is permissible under paragraph 10.02(a) above. The person's written affirmation shall state that he or she has met the standard of conduct necessary for the indemnification under the bylaws. The written undertaking shall provide for repayment of the amount paid or reimbursed by the Ministry if it is ultimately determined that the person has not met the requirements for indemnification. The undertaking shall be an unlimited general obligation of the person, but it need not be secured and it may be accepted without reference to financial ability to make repayment.

11. NOTICES

11.01   Any notice required or permitted by these Bylaws to be given to a director, officer, or member of a committee of the Ministry may be given by mail or email. If mailed, a notice shall be deemed to be delivered when deposited in the United States mail addressed to the person at his or her address as it appears on the records of the Ministry, with postage prepaid. If given by email, a notice shall be deemed to be delivered when sent to the person at his or her email address as it appears on the records of the Ministry. A person may change his or her address or email address by giving written notice to the secretary of the Ministry.

11.02   Whenever any notice is required to be given under the provisions of the Act or under the provisions of the Articles of Incorporation or these Bylaws, a waiver in writing in writing shall signed by a person entitled to receive a notice shall be deemed equivalent to the giving of the notice. A waiver of notice shall be effective whether signed before or after the time stated in the notice being waived.

11.03   The attendance of a person at a meeting shall constitute a waiver of notice of the meeting unless the person attends for the express purpose of objecting to the transaction of any business because the meeting is not lawfully called or convened.

12. SPECIAL PROCEDURES CONCERNING MEETINGS

12.01   The Board of Directors, and any committee of the Ministry may hold a meeting by telephone conference-call procedures or video conference call procedures in which all persons participating in the meeting can hear each other. The notice of a meeting by telephone or video will include all information required to participate in the meeting. Participation of a person in a conference-call meeting constitutes presence of that person at the meeting.

12.02   Any decision required or permitted to be made at a meeting of the Board of Directors, or any committee of the Ministry may be made without a meeting. A decision without a meeting may be made if a written consent to the decision is signed by all of the persons entitled to vote on the matter. The original signed consents shall be placed in the Ministry minute book and kept with the Ministry's records.

12.03   A person who is authorized to exercise a proxy may not exercise the proxy unless the proxy is delivered to the officer presiding at the meeting before the business of the meeting begins. The secretary or other person taking the minutes of the meeting shall record in the minutes the name of the person who executed the proxy and the name of the person authorized to exercise the proxy. If a person who has duly executed a proxy personally attends a meeting, the proxy shall not be effective for that meeting. A proxy filed with the secretary or other designated officer shall remain in force and effect until the first of the following occurs:

> (a) An instrument revoking the proxy is delivered to the secretary or other designated officer.
> (b) The proxy authority expires under the terms of the proxy.
> (c) The proxy authority expires under the terms of the Bylaws.

13. AMENDMENTS TO BYLAWS

These Bylaws may be altered, amended, or repealed, and new or amended bylaws adopted only by the Board of Directors. The notice of any meeting at which the possible amendment, alteration or repeal of these Bylaws or the consideration of new Bylaws is to be discussed shall include the text of the proposed bylaw provisions as well as the text of any existing provisions proposed to be altered, amended or repealed. Alternatively, the notice may include a fair summary of those provisions.

14. MISCELLANEOUS PROVISIONS

14.01   The bylaws shall be construed in accordance with the laws of the State of Texas. All references in the bylaws to statutes, regulations, or other sources of legal authority shall refer to the authorities cited, or their successors, as they may be amended from time to time.

14.02   If any bylaw provision is held to be invalid, illegal, or unenforceable in any respect, the invalidity, illegality, or unenforceability shall not affect any other provision and the bylaws shall be construed as if the invalid, illegal, or unenforceable provision had not been included in the bylaws.

14.03   The headings used in these Bylaws are used for convenience and shall not be considered in construing the terms of the bylaws.

14.04   Wherever the context requires, all words in the bylaws in the male gender shall be deemed to include the female or neuter gender, all singular words shall include the plural, and all plural words shall include the singular.

14.05   The Board of Directors may provide for a corporate seal.

14.06   A person may execute any instrument related to the Ministry by means of a power of attorney if an original executed copy of the power of attorney is provided to the secretary of the Ministry to be kept with the Ministry records.

14.07   The bylaws shall be binding upon and inure to the benefit of the directors, officers, committee members, employees and agents of the Ministry and their respective heirs, executors, administrators, legal representatives, successors, and assigns except as otherwise provided in the bylaws.

14.08 The Ministry is organized and shall be operated exclusively for charitable, educational and religious purposes as defined by Section 501(c)(3) of the Internal Revenue Code, as amended. The Ministry's assets are pledged solely for its use in performing its charitable, educational and religious functions. On discontinuance or dissolution of the Ministry, its assets are to be transferred to another organization, selected by the Ministry's Board of Directors, that qualifies as a tax-exempt organization under Section 501(c)(3) of the Internal Revenue Code, as amended.

CERTIFICATE OF SECRETARY

I certify that I am the duly elected and acting secretary of the Ministry and that the foregoing Bylaws constitute the Bylaws of the Ministry. These Bylaws were duly adopted by the Unanimous Written Consent of the Board of Directors of the Ministry dated June ___, 2014.

DATED: June ____, 2014

By: ____
            Secretary

Unanimous Written Consent
In lieu of an Organizational Meeting of the
Board of Directors
of
Wallace Ministries, Inc.

In accordance with the Texas Non-Profit Corporation Act, as amended (the "Act"), the undersigned, as all the directors of Wallace Ministries, Inc., a Texas corporation (the "Corporation"), hereby adopt the following resolutions to have the same force and effect as if adopted at the organizational meeting of the board of directors of the Corporation, duly called and held under the Act:

Certificate of Formation

RESOLVED, that the Charter of the Corporation having been duly filed in the office of the Secretary of State of the State of Texas on June 2, 2014 is hereby adopted as the Charter of the Corporation and the secretary of the Corporation is instructed to insert a copy of the certificate of formation, as certified by the Secretary of State of Texas, in the minute books of the Corporation.

Bylaws

RESOLVED, that the Bylaws in the form attached hereto, which have been reviewed by the directors of the Corporation, hereby are adopted as the Bylaws of the Corporation, and the secretary of the Corporation is hereby instructed to certify the adoption on a copy of the Bylaws and insert that copy in the minute books of the Corporation.

Officers

RESOLVED, that _________________ is hereby elected as President; _________________ is hereby elected as Vice President and _________________is hereby elected as Secretary/Treasurer, each to serve in these capacity(ies) until the election and qualification of their respective successor.

Organizer's Actions

RESOLVED, that the actions of the organizer of the Corporation, including the election of the initial Board of Directors of the Corporation, taken on behalf of the Corporation, other than any such actions as may have been illegal, tortious, or ultra vires, hereby are ratified and adopted as the actions of the Corporation.

Corporate Seal

RESOLVED, that the seal, if an impression of one is affixed to the margin of this page, hereby is adopted as the seal of the Corporation. If no impression is affixed, the Board may later adopt a Corporate Seal.

Fiscal Year

RESOLVED, that the fiscal year of the Corporation will begin on the first day of January and end on the last day of December of each calendar year.

Bank Accounts

RESOLVED, that the officers of the Corporation hereby are authorized to establish bank accounts in the name and on behalf of the Corporation with any bank, either within or outside the United States, as the officers deem necessary or advisable and, in connection therewith, to execute each bank's regular corporate resolution forms, which are incorporated by reference in and made a part of this resolution, and that the secretary hereby is directed to place a copy of each corporate resolution form so executed in the minute books of the Corporation;

RESOLVED FURTHER, that the president of the Corporation be the authorized signatory on any bank accounts established in the name and on behalf of the Corporation;

RESOLVED FURTHER, that the president of the Corporation is hereby authorized (1) to designate any other employee or officer of the Corporation as an authorized signatory on any bank account established in the name and on behalf of the Corporation, if the president deems the designation necessary or advisable, and in connection with that designation (2) to establish limitations on the authority of the designated signatory, including amounts or requirements for cosigners; and

RESOLVED FURTHER, that the secretary or any assistant secretary of the Corporation, when requested by the president, will certify the adoption of these resolutions to any bank in which an account is established, together with a certificate of incumbency naming the persons then holding the offices of the Corporation.

Organization Expenses

RESOLVED, that the officers of the Corporation hereby are directed to pay all expenses properly incurred in connection with the organization of the Corporation.

Books and Records

RESOLVED, that the secretary of the Corporation hereby is instructed to purchase any record books, books of account, checks, stationery, or office supplies necessary or appropriate for the proper administration of the affairs of the Corporation.

Foreign Qualification

RESOLVED, that for the purpose of authorizing the Corporation to do business in any state or territory of the United States or any foreign country necessary for the Corporation to transact business, the officers of the Corporation hereby are authorized to appoint and substitute all necessary agents or attorneys for the service of process to execute, for and on behalf of the Corporation, all necessary certificates, reports, powers of attorney, and other such instruments as may be required by the laws of the state, territory, or country to authorize the Corporation to transact business therein and, whenever it is necessary for the Corporation to cease doing business and withdraw therefrom, (1) to revoke any appointment of agent or attorney for service of process and to file any certificates, reports, revocation of appointment, or surrender of authority necessary to terminate the authority of the Corporation to do business in any state, territory, or country; and (2) to execute all general corporate resolution forms that may be required to effect any of the foregoing, the resolution forms being hereby incorporated by reference and made a part of this resolution; and the secretary of the Corporation hereby is directed to place a copy of each corporate resolution form so executed in the minute books of the Corporation.

Conflict of Interest Policy

RESOLVED, that the Conflict of Interest Policy is the form attached hereto is hereby adopted as the policy of the Corporation.

General Authority

RESOLVED, that the officers of the Corporation hereby are authorized and directed on behalf of the Corporation to execute and deliver all other instruments, documents, and certificates, to pay all costs, fees, and taxes, and to take all other actions as may be in their judgment necessary, proper, or advisable to carry out and comply with the purposes and intent of the foregoing resolutions; and that all the actions of the officers of the Corporation that are consistent with the purposes and intent of these resolutions are in all respects hereby approved, ratified, confirmed, and adopted as the actions of the Corporation.

IN WITNESS WHEREOF, each member of the Board of Directors of the Corporation has executed this Unanimous Written Consent in one or more counterparts, each of which shall be deemed to be one and the same instrument, as of the date first above written.

____

Board Member

____

Board Member

____

Board Member

____

Board Member

____

Board Member

Conflict of Interest Policy
Of
Wallace Ministries, Inc.

Article I
Purpose

The purpose of the conflict of interest policy is to protect the interest of Wallace Ministries, Inc. (the "Ministry") when it is contemplating entering into a transaction or arrangement that might benefit the private interest of an officer or director of the Ministry or might result in a possible excess benefit transaction. This policy is intended to supplement but not replace any applicable state and federal laws governing conflict of interest applicable to nonprofit and charitable organizations.

Article II
Definitions

1. Interested Person
Any director, principal officer, or member of a committee with governing board delegated powers, who has a direct or indirect financial interest, as defined below, is an interested person.

2. Financial Interest
A person has a financial interest if the person has, directly or indirectly, through business, investment, or family:
a. An ownership or investment interest in any entity with which the Ministry has a transaction or arrangement,
b. A compensation arrangement with the Ministry or with any entity or individual with which the Ministry has a transaction or arrangement, or
c. A potential ownership or investment interest in, or compensation arrangement with, any entity or individual with which the Ministry is

negotiating a transaction or arrangement.

Compensation includes direct and indirect remuneration as well as gifts or favors that are not insubstantial. A financial interest is not necessarily a conflict of interest. Under Article III, Section 2, a person who has a financial interest may have a conflict of interest only if the appropriate governing board or committee decides that a conflict of interest exists.

Article III
Procedures

1. **Duty to Disclose**
In connection with any actual or possible conflict of interest, an interested person must disclose the existence of the financial interest and be given the opportunity to disclose all material facts to the directors and members of committees with governing board delegated powers considering the proposed transaction or arrangement.

2. **Determining Whether a Conflict of Interest Exists**
After disclosure of the financial interest and all material facts, and after any discussion with the interested person, he/she shall leave the governing board or committee meeting while the determination of a conflict of interest is discussed and voted upon. The remaining board or committee members shall decide if a conflict of interest exists.

3. **Procedures for Addressing the Conflict of Interest**
a. An interested person may make a presentation at the governing board or committee meeting, but after the presentation, he/she shall leave the meeting during the discussion of, and the vote on, the transaction or arrangement involving the possible conflict of interest.
b. The chairperson of the governing board or committee shall, if appropriate, appoint a disinterested person or committee to investigate alternatives to the proposed transaction or arrangement.
c. After exercising due diligence, the governing board or committee shall determine whether the Ministry can obtain with reasonable efforts a more advantageous transaction or arrangement from a person or entity that would not give rise to a conflict of interest.
d. If a more advantageous transaction or arrangement is not reasonably

possible under circumstances not producing a conflict of interest, the governing board or committee shall determine by a majority vote of the disinterested directors whether the transaction or arrangement is in the Ministry's best interest, for its own benefit, and whether it is fair and reasonable. In conformity with the above determination it shall make its decision as to whether to enter into the transaction or arrangement.

4. **Violations of the Conflicts of Interest Policy**
a. If the governing board or committee has reasonable cause to believe a member has failed to disclose actual or possible conflicts of interest, it shall inform the member of the basis for such belief and afford the member an opportunity to explain the alleged failure to disclose.
b. If, after hearing the member's response and after making further investigation as warranted by the circumstances, the governing board or committee determines the member has failed to disclose an actual or possible conflict of interest, it shall take appropriate disciplinary and corrective action.

Article IV
Records of Proceedings

The minutes of the governing board and all committees with board delegated powers shall contain:
a. The names of the persons who disclosed or otherwise were found to have a financial interest in connection with an actual or possible conflict of interest, the nature of the financial interest, any action taken to determine whether a conflict of interest was present, and the governing board's or committee's decision as to whether a conflict of interest in fact existed.
b. The names of the persons who were present for discussions and votes relating to the transaction or arrangement, the content of the discussion, including any alternatives to the proposed transaction or arrangement, and a record of any votes taken in connection with the proceedings.

Article V
Compensation

a. A voting member of the governing board who receives compensation, directly or indirectly, from the Ministry for services is precluded from voting on matters pertaining to that member's compensation.

b. A voting member of any committee whose jurisdiction includes compensation matters and who receives compensation, directly or indirectly, from the Ministry for services is precluded from voting on matters pertaining to that member's compensation.

c. No voting member of the governing board or any committee whose jurisdiction includes compensation matters and who receives compensation, directly or indirectly, from the Ministry, either individually or collectively, is prohibited from providing information to any committee regarding compensation.

Article VI
Annual Statements

Each director, principal officer and member of a committee with governing board delegated powers shall annually sign a statement which affirms such person:

a. Has received a copy of the conflicts of interest policy,

b. Has read and understands the policy,

c. Has agreed to comply with the policy, and

d. Understands the Ministry is charitable and in order to maintain its federal tax exemption it must engage primarily in activities which accomplish one or more of its tax-exempt purposes.

Article VII
Periodic Reviews

To ensure the Ministry operates in a manner consistent with charitable purposes and does not engage in activities that could jeopardize its tax-exempt status, periodic reviews shall be conducted. The periodic reviews shall, at a minimum, include the following subjects:

a. Whether compensation arrangements and benefits are reasonable, based on competent survey information, and the result of arm's length bargaining.

b. Whether partnerships, joint ventures, and arrangements with management conform to the Ministry's written policies, are properly recorded, reflect reasonable investment or payments for goods and services, further charitable purposes and do not result in inurement, impermissible private benefit or in an excess benefit transaction.

Article VIII
Use of Outside Experts

When conducting the periodic reviews as provided for in Article VII, the Ministry may, but need not, use outside advisors. If outside experts are used, their use shall not relieve the governing board of its responsibility for ensuring periodic reviews are conducted.

CERTIFICATE OF SECRETARY

I certify that I am the duly elected and acting secretary of the Ministry and that the foregoing Conflict of Interest Policy constitutes the Conflict of Interest Policy of the Ministry. This Conflict of Interest Policy was duly adopted by the Unanimous Written Consent of the Board of Directors of the Ministry dated June ___, 2014.

DATED: June ____, 2014

By: ____
        Secretary

www.ingramcontent.com/pod-product-compliance
Lightning Source LLC
Chambersburg PA
CBHW031810150726
47989CB00006B/2943